NO
MORE
CARBS
CONFUSION.

A straightforward manual for understanding carbs and adjusting your intake.

Jim C. Bernard

Copyright © 2023 by Jim C. Bernard

All rights reserved. No portion of this book may be duplicated or communicated in any way, whether electronically or mechanically, including by photocopying, recording, or information storing or retrieval systems, without the author's or their representatives' prior written consent.

CONTENTS.

INTRODUCTION.

Does the word "carbs" give you the chills? People are truly perplexed by the myths and truths surrounding carbohydrates, such as "no carbs before night" and "carbs make you fat." With so many deceptive illusions about carbs floating around, it's understandable why many are turning to the keto diet, avoiding carbs before night, and believing that all carbohydrates are unhealthy (they aren't).

It's time to dispel the myths that we have previously heard.

Your body uses carbohydrates as its primary energy source. The body switches to burning fat as fuel when carbohydrates aren't being consumed and your glycogen stores are low. Your body strongly favors using carbohydrates as fuel, which is why ketosis is a survival mechanism.

Carbs are good for the body. They provide energy for your body's muscles, neurological system, and red blood cells. Additionally, they stop the protein from being used as fuel. This is still another benefit, as our body prefers to use protein for tissue growth and repair rather than for fuel.

Our bodies can run on the energy that comes from carbohydrates. When you consume food that contains carbohydrates, your body converts those carbohydrates into glucose. " The main fuel that constantly circulates in our blood is glucose. It serves as the brain's primary source of fuel.

It's critical to realize that everyone's reaction to carbohydrate ingestion varies. Start with nutritious, complex carbs first, and then determine how much you believe is appropriate for your particular genetic composition.

Carbs can be highly nourishing and good for our health and performance, in the end. The key to making a difference for you is to focus on the quality of the carbohydrates rather than their quantity.

Good and Bad Carbohydrates.

How can one differentiate between healthy and unhealthy carbohydrates? Understanding the types of carbohydrates we consume is crucial because they affect how the body processes them. Carbohydrates that are whole and unprocessed are viewed as healthy. Sweet potatoes, bananas, potatoes, brown rice, yucca, lentils, and dates are a few examples. All of these foods are still full of nutrients and have just undergone minor modifications that don't compromise their nutritional worth.

Carbohydrates that have been refined remove their fiber content. They have undergone changes that cause the food to lose numerous essential vitamins, minerals, and fatty acids during processing. Fruit drinks, white flour, white rice, and white pasta are examples of refined carbohydrates.

How many healthy carbohydrates should I eat?

How many grams of carbohydrates you need each day is one of the most often asked questions about carbohydrates. To begin with, I want to stress that everyone's carb demands vary depending on a variety of factors, including age, sex, body type, degree of exercise and training, and metabolic health. A range of 100-150 grams of healthy carbs is excellent for most people who are trying to lose weight to support energy levels and general vigor. This translates to a range of 15% to 30% of total calories coming from healthy carbohydrates.

Only those who are serious athletes or fitness lovers would be the few exceptions. They typically need more carbohydrates for hormone support, muscle protein synthesis, and recuperation. These people would need 150–250 grams of carbohydrates per day.

On the opposite end of the spectrum, those who have metabolic problems like type 2 diabetes or Alzheimer's disease tend to favor a low-carb diet, which is particularly successful in treating diabetes and other neurological conditions. They should take in 60 to 90 grams of carbohydrates each day. Even some people have a sensitivity to carbohydrates. The inability to adequately digest and absorb carbohydrates is indicated by the absence of certain digestive enzymes such as lactase, amylase, maltase, sucrase, and isomaltase.

CHAPTER ONE.

Why the current diet and health strategy is ineffective.

Nearly all people who have attempted to reduce weight have experienced the bitter pill of failure. That sensation you have when, despite your best efforts to stay with your diet and exercise regimen long enough to see results, you are unable to achieve your goals of being healthier, fitting into sexier clothes, or moving through life (and into airplane seats) with more ease and comfort.

Almost everyone around someone who is struggling to lose weight tends to blame themselves. In actuality, a sizable percentage of medical professionals view obesity as a personal shortcoming. However, this viewpoint reveals an utter disregard for human physiology and how it affects weight reduction.

In reality, most diets fail because the body triggers several strong physiological mechanisms that help to protect us from losing too much excess weight. Many of these mechanisms are brought on by changes in the hypothalamus, which is situated at the base of the brain.

These mechanisms have been essential to our species' survival because they stop weight loss from continuing and encourage weight increase. The majority of human history occurred before agricultural times, during which food availability was largely seasonal and irregular. Survival during the lean season was guaranteed through energy conservation.

According to research, even after reducing weight, people frequently have trouble keeping it off.

Researchers from a variety of disciplines, including nutrition, psychology, and physiology, have evaluated a range of various diets in short- and long-term settings during the past few decades. Additionally, while it is simple to find individual studies that support a particular diet (which explains why books, blogs, and articles claim that a certain diet has "been shown" to do a certain thing), a thorough analysis of the data reveals that there is no one weight loss diet that is superior to another for the majority of people.

So why is it so difficult for so many people to lose weight permanently?

First of all, given the environment and conditions in which we live, our bodies are not designed to make weight loss simple.

The problem of weight gain following weight reduction was the topic of a panel discussion organized by the National Institutes of Health in 2014, which focused on the biological, environmental, and behavioral variables that can make long-term weight loss so challenging. According to the panel, after weight reduction, the body undergoes a series of physiological changes that lower the number of calories it burns, demanding further calorie reduction to maintain weight loss. But it gets harder and harder to cut calories as the brain adjusts to losing weight. Why? The brain's reaction to calorie reduction usually involves increasing desires for highly rewarding foods (tasty food that's a combination of sweet, fatty, and salty), while simultaneously decreasing our experience of fullness. In other words, our body and brain actively support weight regain while fiercely defending against weight loss. It's a never-ending "feedback loop," and it's exceedingly challenging to correct the loop once it veers off course.

The Connotative Sense of "Diet".

Let's be clear: the phrase "diet" generally connotes restrictive eating, and this strategy frequently serves as a springboard for the emergence of disordered eating behaviors. But when we overeat, exercise little, and gain weight, our natural response is to limit our intake and exercise more.

In fact, at any given time, approximately 100 million Americans are dieting. [2]

Unfortunately, once we start to limit our calorie intake, our hunger intensifies and we find ourselves in a struggle between wanting to eat to meet our body's all-consuming requirements and yet not wanting to eat to avoid gaining weight. Dieting is believed to be the solution to weight management.

The Reason Diets Fail.

Dieting is an action that cannot be sustained, which is why diets fail. The majority of people who diet usually end up gaining back the weight they lost plus more. Additionally, a lot of people are on diets without even realizing it. Some diets are simple to avoid because they have their names in the titles of books; examples include paleo, keto, and others. The issue is that modern diets tend to be covert. Despite being unachievable, they pass for "healthy lifestyle programs." You should have reached your target weight by now if dieting worked.

The Effects of Diets on the Body.

You would anticipate seeing some results from all the time, effort, and mental energy you put into dieting. Many people do lose weight, but two to five years later, the majority of them gain it back.

This could be a result of the chemical changes that can occur in your body when you diet by counting calories, which can make it more difficult to maintain weight loss. According to studies, ghrelin, sometimes known as the "hunger hormone," is produced at a higher rate than leptin, the "satiety hormone." It may still be difficult to maintain your new weight even after you reach your desired weight and stop dieting since you may continue to feel more hungry than before. And you could even discover that food tastes better than it did before you started dieting! It is caused by these biological changes. It is challenging to maintain good intentions due to these physiologic changes.

Additionally, dieting can cause you to crave the items you are supposed to avoid. When you're given a list of items you're not allowed to eat, you frequently crave them more, just like a kid when they're told they can't. Additionally, if you indulge in these off-limits meals, you can feel out of control because you don't know when you'll be able to do so again

What should I do now that I've abandoned the diet?

The good thing is that you don't have to give up 95% of your life to lose 5% of your weight, and you can be healthy without dieting. The steps are as follows:

Monitor your hunger.
Your appetite is a built-in system for controlling your weight. A non-diet method enables you to reconnect with your hunger, a natural biological

cue, whereas dieting teaches us to avoid or fear hunger. Because they fill your mind with rules and limits, diets make it difficult to eat instinctively and pay attention to your body's inherent guidance.

Eat just when you're truly hungry and quit when you're satisfied. Check in with your body. While some people feel better eating three larger meals each day, others prefer eating six smaller meals throughout the day. Regaining awareness of your hunger signals and appetite will help you choose what works best for you.

Use health as your motivation rather than weight Loss.

Do you participate in this new healthy exercise to feel better or to lose weight? You might be more prone to slacking off if you're forming new behaviors just for the sake of slimming down. Weight loss is rarely linear and frequently requires more time than we are told. When you adopt healthy new behaviors to lose weight, you might be tempted to stop doing them if you don't see the weight reduction you were hoping for or if you temporarily gain it (this can happen). On the other hand, if you aim to feel well and powerful, you'll be more resilient when your weight doesn't track as you'd like it to.

Demonstrate crowding.

Most diets contain a list of off-limits things, which makes you inevitably crave those meals. In its place, I advise "crowding." Concentrate on eating more whole grains, fruit, vegetables, and legumes. You won't feel deprived if you consume more nutritious foods since they will naturally drive out the less nutritious ones. Stock your refrigerator with nutritious foods and discover quick, delectable recipes to prepare them.

Avoid all-or-nothing strategies.

For the majority of us, eliminating entire food groups—for instance, giving up sugar or avoiding carbohydrates—is not sustainable. Do you want to go your entire life without ever having pasta or baked cheesecake? While on a diet, you might be content to temporarily abstain from these indulgences, but ultimately you'll long to enjoy them once more. A new birthday, family meal, long weekend, holiday, wedding, office party, or Christmas function is always around the corner. It is better to have a moderate stance. By preparing more nutrient-dense meals at home, including more vegetables in recipes, and actively savoring your meals, you can eat more healthfully.

Regain your joy.

It feels simple to perform an activity when you enjoy it. It feels more like a decision than like a punishment. Your new, healthy habits won't last long if they feel like a job; doing them will take too much willpower. Find an activity that you genuinely enjoy if going to the gym sounds painful to you. Yoga or dance, perhaps. While engaging in your favorite hobbies may not result in as much energy loss as going to the gym or running, you are much more likely to stick with them since you enjoy them. Consistency is ultimately the secret to excellent health. And delight is the secret of perseverance.

CHAPTER TWO.

Introduction to Carbs and Carbs Control.

When you consume meals or beverages containing carbohydrates, also referred to as "carbs," your body converts them into glucose (a form of sugar), which then increases the level of glucose in your blood. That glucose is used as fuel by your body to keep you moving throughout the day. This is what you most likely refer to as your "blood sugar" or "blood glucose." The carbohydrates you consume are crucial in treating diabetes. The pancreas discharges insulin to assist the cells in absorbing glucose after the body converts turns those carbohydrates into glucose.

Hyperglycemia is the medical term for when a person's blood glucose—or blood sugar—is too high. One reason for "highs" is that there is insufficient insulin in your body to digest the additional glucose in the blood or your body's cells fail to respond to the insulin that is released, causing extra glucose to build up. The clinical word for low blood sugar is hypoglycemia. Sometimes "lows" are brought on by inadequate carbohydrate intake or a pharmaceutical imbalance. In essence, the amount of carbs we eat affects our blood sugar, thus balancing is essential!

Starches, sugar, and fiber are the three main forms of carbohydrates found in food. The term "total carbohydrate" refers to all three of these kinds of carbohydrates, as you can see on the nutrition labels for the food you purchase. The idea is to select carbohydrates that are nutrient-dense, meaning they are high in fiber, vitamins, and minerals and low in added sugars, sodium, and bad fats. Choosing carbohydrate-containing foods:

Eat as much of these unprocessed, non-starchy, whole vegetables as you can. Because they include more fiber than carbohydrates, non-starchy veggies like lettuce, cucumbers, broccoli, tomatoes, and green beans have less of an influence on your blood sugar. Keep in mind that you should have these on half of your plate.

Consume a few of these: whole, barely processed carbohydrate items. These foods, which are known as starchy carbs, include fruits like apples, blueberries, strawberries, and melons; whole, unprocessed grains; starchy vegetables; and beans and lentils such as black beans, kidney beans, chickpeas, and green lentils. The foods in this category should make up a quarter of your plate.

Reduce your consumption of refined, highly processed, and sugar-added carbohydrate items. These include refined grains like white bread, and white rice, sugary cereal, sugary drinks like soda, sweet tea, and juice, and sweets and snack items like cake, cookies, candies, and chips.

It's crucial to keep in mind that we rarely consume carbohydrates alone unless we're eating a processed item, like a lollipop or soft drink. Most generally, food is a combination of many nutrients. Instead of using the individual nutrients separately, we develop a healthy eating pattern using the combination of nutrients in the complete food. Even when choosing whole foods, we may still consume more energy than our bodies require because we spend a large portion of our days sitting and not moving about. In actuality, the cause of our ill health is excess carbohydrate consumption compared to what the body requires. A high metabolic load is imposed on the body by consuming too many carbohydrates. Over time, the body is forced to deal with high blood sugar levels, which are the result of digesting food's sugar and starch. This causes weight increase, poor metabolism, and a high risk of heart disease.

Here are 10 red flags that indicate you've been ingesting too many carbohydrates:

1. Gaining weight
2. A high sugar level
3. Tiredness
4. High triglycerides
5. High insulin levels
6. Skin problems
High Triglyceride Levels
8. Having a sweet tooth
9. Bloating and diarrhea

10. Disturbances to the digestive system occur.

There are many reasons why people might decide to cut back on their carbohydrate intake. People with type 2 diabetes should make an effort to strike a balance between the need to consume enough carbs to provide energy and the need to consume fewer carbohydrates to control blood sugar levels. Others aim to limit their intake of carbohydrates to maintain a balanced diet that includes more nutritious items. Whatever the cause, several methods can be employed to ensure that the reduction in carbohydrates yields the desired benefits without causing a loss of vital nutrients.

Smart Methods to Reduce Carbohydrates Intake.

1. Avoid drinking alcoholic or sweetened beverages, and limit your intake of juice. Sugar, a carbohydrate, and calories can be found in relatively high concentrations in sodas, sweet tea, juices, and alcoholic beverages. Juice also seems healthy, but it contains a lot of sugar

because the fruit's fiber, which keeps you full for longer, has been removed. Instead, stick to eating the fruit itself, which offers a more gradual release of carbohydrates and longer-lasting energy.

2. Examine foods for hidden sugars. Check the food label for "added sugar" by reading it. The better number is one digit, and the lower the better. Over 10% of your daily calories from added sugar should be avoided. You should limit your added sugar intake to 45 grams per day, for instance, if your daily calorie goal is 1,800. Many meals, including those we consider to be healthy, like yogurt, contain added sugars. Some yogurts with added sugar have more sugar than ice cream.

3. Whenever possible, choose whole grains. When compared to processed grains, whole grains are higher in fiber and nutrients like iron and B vitamins, which might make you feel fuller longer after eating carbohydrates. For example, start your day with a high-fiber breakfast cereal. To ensure you are indeed

consuming a whole grain, look for the word "whole" in the first or main ingredient.

4. Be mindful of serving sizes. About 1/3 cup of cooked pasta or rice, 1 cup of milk, 4 to 6 crackers, 1/2 cup of a starchy vegetable, like potatoes, or a piece of fruit the size of a tennis ball should make up a portion of carbohydrates. Managing our portion sizes can be made easier by using smaller plates, bowls, and cups.

5. Instead of frying, use the broiler and bake. Avoid battering and frying meats and vegetables when cooking them. The flour that was used to make the coating is loaded with extra carbohydrates that your body does not require. When broiling, use a lot of herbs and spices to enhance the flavor. When baking chicken or fish, use an egg batter and crushed bran flakes combination for a crispy exterior.

CHAPTER THREE.

Glucose and Insulin.

Your body naturally produces a specific quantity of insulin each time you eat something. Your body produces insulin continuously if you regularly eat and snack.

Important quick note: Your body does not burn fat when it is creating insulin!

This means that when you consume a lot of carbohydrates, your body is told to turn the blood glucose into fat.

In other words, the body pursues its goal of storing fat with greater zeal the higher your insulin levels are.

Your cells may respond to insulin less effectively in the long run as a result of this. They start to resist. In this situation, blood glucose levels are still high and your pancreas is struggling to produce enough insulin. Your health may suffer as a result, which is very serious.

Insulin is the main hormone involved in fat accumulation and weight gain and is released in response to blood glucose levels. Although insulin is frequently associated with diabetes, it is a major factor in weight growth for everyone, regardless of whether they have diabetes, and must be controlled to successfully maintain a healthy weight.

The primary anabolic hormone in our bodies, insulin encourages "growing" rather than "breaking down" in the body (e.g., the storage of fat). When there is too much glucose in the blood, insulin instructs cells to store it for later use. We must manage our insulin to tell the body to burn fat rather than carbs because losing weight typically necessitates burning through fat storage.

Increased insulin levels tell the liver and muscles to store excess glucose as chains of glycogen as there's more glucose in the blood than what the body requires to meet energy needs. Once the muscles and liver are full of glycogen, any extra glucose is converted to fat (triglycerides) and transmitted through the blood to be deposited in fat cells throughout the body. You can conceive of the liver and muscle as having limited, short-term energy storage in the form of glycogen, whereas fat cells have virtually infinite, long-term energy storage in the form of triglycerides.

When we aren't eating—whether we are fasting, between meals, or sleeping—the lack of dietary glucose raises our insulin levels.

The Value Of Recognizing And Managing Our Glucose Levels.

At Levels, we think the secret to success is understanding precisely how your body reacts to certain nutrients. Fortunately, insulin responses and glucose levels frequently coincide. Knowing how much food elevates blood sugar helps us forecast how much insulin our body will be exposed to, which helps us determine whether our body is more likely to be burning fat or storing it.

After reading this, you might conclude that the best way to reduce insulin and lose fat and weight is to consume relatively few carbohydrates and a diet high in fat. Even though this might be a piece of the puzzle, it is not the only one. It's crucial to keep in mind that many complex carbs and lean protein sources can support our bodies' optimal functioning without necessarily causing large rises in blood sugar or insulin levels.

How Glucose Tracking Can Guide Our Efforts to Lose Weight.

Everything begins with the glucose levels; as they rise, insulin is usually released. Increased insulin levels cause fat to be stored as body weight. Insulin resistance is a condition in which our cells lose their sensitivity to insulin over time if blood glucose levels are continuously increased as a result of diet and insulin production is active all the time. As a result, our baseline insulin levels rise because we require more and more circulating insulin to deliver glucose into cells. This procedure directly undermines attempts to lose weight.

High insulin levels in obese people also cause "leptin resistance" and decreased leptin signaling, which makes it difficult for us to feel full and more likely that we will continue consuming calories instead of burning stored fat for energy. On the other side, reduced

insulin levels result in reduced glucose levels, which cause weight loss and a reduction in the mass of fat in the body.
Other substances besides insulin cause fat storage.

You are well aware that insulin makes fat cells absorb fatty acids and glucose. There's also another justification for the claim that it makes people acquire weight.

Hormone-sensitive lipase (HSL), an enzyme found in your fat cells, aids in the breakdown of body fat into fatty acids for burning. Insulin is thought to further encourage weight gain by suppressing HSL function.
The fact that dietary fat also inhibits HSL and that your body doesn't require a lot of insulin to store dietary fat as body fat is something that those who dislike carbs and insulin prefer to disregard.
 This is why eating as much dietary fat as you desire won't automatically result in weight loss. And the reason why the study has found that eating carbs and fats separately has no impact

on weight loss (eating carbs and fats combined has no impact either way).

It all boils down to maintaining a healthy energy balance; if you consistently provide your body with more energy than it can burn, whether, in the form of protein, carbohydrates, or fat, you'll gain weight.

Insulin Is Not the Issue... Being sedentary and overweight is.

In conclusion, carbohydrate intake and insulin levels are as follows:

Regularly consuming significant amounts of carbohydrates will eventually lead to issues if you are overweight and inactive. You'll experience increasing insulin resistance in your body, which may eventually result in Type 2 diabetes, and you'll be more susceptible to heart disease.

You'll never have these issues if you maintain a healthy weight, engage in regular exercise, and consume at least a moderately sane diet. Your body will continue to be sensitive to insulin and be able to utilize the carbs you consume.

CHAPTER FOUR.

What is Carbs Threshold/Tolerance?

The daily carbohydrate intake that enables one to achieve their health and weight loss goals while experiencing vitality, stable energy, decent sleep, tranquility, and clarity of mind is known as a carb threshold.

Are you aware that several recalcitrant health issues could be caused by your carb threshold: High blood pressure with weight gain, particularly if you are having trouble losing weight or are not seeing results from your usual weight-loss methods, may indicate that you have developed a sensitivity to carbohydrates. This indicates that fewer carbohydrates are required to increase your insulin levels. Consider it in this way. You could probably have eaten anything in your younger years, let's say in college or your early 20s, and your weight wouldn't change. Now, the scale scarcely moves when you diet and are very focused on cutting out sweets, bread, and other delicacies. How come? because over time, your cells have gotten less sensitive to glucose. Additionally, insulin serves as the messenger hormone that instructs your cells to absorb glucose after meals. To get the glucose into the cells, the insulin has to speak louder as you grow less receptive to the message (as a result of overuse). In essence, your sensitivity to glucose and carbs has decreased. Protein and fat have less of an impact on blood sugar than carbohydrates do.

Your body's natural point of equilibrium, or the weight at which you don't lose or gain any more weight, is determined by your carbohydrate tolerance. Numerous variables, such as age, level of fitness, amount of exercise, and others, affect this number. The average person's range of net carbohydrates per day will be between 40 and 120 grams, but some people who have a very hard time losing or maintaining weight may find that their range is considerably greater. Do not forget that these are ranges.

Your range expands as you increase your activity and exercise.

Why is it important to understand your unique carb tolerance?

You must discover how many grams of Net Carbs you can eat each day without gaining weight if you want to maintain your ideal weight once you've reached it.

How can you determine your carbohydrate tolerance?

During Pre-Maintenance, when you may need to "play about" within a 10-gram range to continue the process of dropping the final few pounds, you start to gain a handle on your carb tolerance. You are officially in Lifetime Maintenance when you reach your target weight and maintain it for a month. At that point, you will know how to eat for the rest of your life. This is what we mean by your personal carb tolerance/threshold.

Will my carb tolerance stay the same after I figure it out?

No, not always. Your carb tolerance may drop as you get older and less active, or it may rise if you decide to become more active. Your carb tolerance may also be affected by changes in medication dosage or the start of menopause.

CONCLUSION.

The type of carbohydrate you decide to consume is important since some sources are healthier than others. The type of carbohydrates in the diet is more significant than their quantity, whether high or low. Example, grains like quinoa, rye, barley, and whole wheat bread are healthier substitutes than French fries or highly processed white bread.

A high number of people are confused about carbs, but it's necessary to remember that eating carbohydrates from nutritious and healthy meals is more crucial than adhering to a strict diet that restricts or counts the grams of carbohydrates taken.

More so than focusing on or avoiding a specific nutrient, a well-balanced diet that includes unprocessed carbohydrates, adequate sleep, and physical activity is likely to promote good health and healthy body weight.

There is evidence that consuming a lot of fruits, vegetables, and whole grains can help with weight management. Their bulk and fiber content make you feel satiated on fewer calories, which helps with weight control. Contrary to what proponents of low-carb diets assert, few studies demonstrate a link between a diet high in healthy carbohydrates and weight gain or obesity. A balanced diet must include carbohydrates since they are an important source of numerous vital elements. Regardless, not all carbohydrates are healthy for you.

Decide on your carbohydrates carefully. Limit meals like sugary drinks, pastries, and confectionery that include added sugars and processed grains. These are low in nutrition yet high in calories. Fruits, veggies, and whole grains are better choices instead.

www.ingramcontent.com/pod-product-compliance
Lightning Source LLC
Chambersburg PA
CBHW061558250726

48657CB00021B/2329